So You've Had A Stroke (2nd Ed.)

by

Maxwell R Watson

Or

How to Avoid a Stroke

ISBN: 13: 9781511707176

Published at Createspace.com

And at

www.smashwords.com
max@maxwellrwatson.com

Dedication

I dedicate this book to my longsuffering wife Christine, you are amazing darling; and I love you more than I can ever find words to say.

Disclaimer

I am not attempting to answer every possible question anyone could have, that is simply not possible. Nor am I addressing issues you should not discuss with your own doctor or therapists'. Nor am I some kind of font of all wisdom, because I'm not, I'm just a guy who survived a massive stroke and who wants to encourage other people in that situation to keep going, life is worth living. In addition, I want to encourage all people that are brain injury free to do whatever you need to do to stay that way. If you are a ultra busy professional, stop, take a life inventory, make whatever changes that need to be made to ensure you are healthy, your BMI is under 30 and you are not a walking stroke or heart attack.

Human Brain Facts

1. No pain. There are no pain receptors in the brain, so the brain itself, can feel no pain.
2. Blood vessels. There are 160,000 kilometres of blood vessels in the brain.
3. Fat. The human brain is the fattest organ in the body and may consist of at least 60% fat.
4. Skin. Your skin weighs twice as much as your brain.
5. Water. The brain contains about 75% water.
6. Grey matter. The brain's grey matter is made up of neurons, which gather and transmit signals.
7. Your brain consists of about 100 billion neurons.
8. There are anywhere from 1,000 to 10,000 synapses for each neuron.

Avoiding a stoke

I begin this 2nd edition by some words on avoiding stroke.

How to avoid a stroke:

It is very simple folks:

1. Get your BMI, Body Mass index to be, not just safe, but correct. There are many online BMI checkers, Google it and take your pick. Do not think you can cheat by lowering your real weight. You are, as my old high school science teacher was fond of saying, only fooling yourself. A calculator won't be impressed if you lie. Be honest and work at whatever it takes to get that weight/fat ratio right for your age and height.

2. Eat well, correctly and well balanced.

3. Do not overwork. If you are a workaholic, get help to get your work/life balance to a healthy balance.

You may think I am being over dramatic, I'm not. Stroke is NOT funny, and is NOT something to ignore.

I know. I survived a massive stroke in May 2004. No-one wants to go through this torture if it can be avoided and some 80% of strokes are preventable. Following those three points above could well save your life. If you have what is often termed a mini stroke, more correctly a TIA (A transient ischaemic attack). Then insist your Doctor/s take action. I had two TIA's but my GP was either too busy or ignorant and did nothing. So when I suffered the major stroke I was not "protected" by and preventive medication.

Furthermore my main advice is this: do whatever it takes to avoid a stroke.

Introduction

"When you get into a tight place and everything goes against you, till it seems as though you could not hang on a minute longer, never give up then, for that is just the place and time that the tide will turn."

Harriet Beecher Stowe

I am going to assume that you, or someone close to you, has suffered a stroke! Firstly, I would like to say that I am truly sorry about that. Secondly, I did too; and no, I do not have all the answers for you or anyone. I simply wanted to be able to give people a free resource to help in this difficult time. You probably have, or soon will have, dozens of questions. I would also highly advise that you contact your local or regional Brain Injury Association for assistance and further information.

I have written this booklet in an attempt to help you understand some of what you have experienced and are experiencing. However, the number one positive thing is that you had survived and you have a life yet to live, enjoy and succeed in.

You may not think that surviving a Stroke is necessarily the best thing in all this but I assure you that it is, and a whole lot better than the other option. If you are a relative, of a Stroke survivor you need to understand many things will now possibly change and I will address some of these issues as I proceed.

I have chosen to ask and answer questions that I had and sadly had to find out for myself.

1stly

You will have lots of doctors and therapists telling you many things about yourself that will be very difficult for you to understand and indeed to accept.

You have an injury (called an acquired brain injury or **ABI**) to your brain and this will mean that things are now different for you or your loved one.

The level or amount of these differences depends entirely on the area of your brain that has been affected and the amount of damage there is to that affected area. Doctors will tell you many things, but ultimately they do not know if you totally recover or not. The brain is the most complicated organ in the mortal body, and it has abilities far beyond any current human understanding to make new pathways (that's called neuroplasticity). To read more on neuroplasticity go to

http://en.wikipedia.org/wiki/Neuroplasticity

It is going to take you time to understand the full impact of your Stroke. That's OK, no one has the right to tell you things like: "get over it," "just accept the way you are and make the most your life" and other hurtful and meaningless statements that people sometimes make. We each need to take the time we need to come to terms with surviving a Stroke and what that means to you, and that is different for every single person.

You may well have times of depression because of the affects on your life. I sure did. Just remember **DO NOT** isolate yourself and **DO NOT** make major decisions when in a depressed state.

If you realize you are depressed see your doctor **immediately**, DO NOT attempt to use other people's prescribed medication, over the counter herbal medicine, illegal drugs or alcohol to "help you get by" or "cope" – They **do not** work and in most cases will only make matters far, far worse.

If you feel like it would be better to have died than survive. Seek help you could well be depressed and in need of help. By the way, those thoughts though appearing real, are in fact a lie. Life is good and in time you will learn how to take full advantage of the time you have to engage in life, family, friends and fun once again.

HOW WILL MY LIFE CHANGE?

This will depend entirely on the extent of any disability you may have following your time in rehabilitation.

You may have to relearn how to do many normal everyday things in order to live an independent life. I had to relearn how to many things myself, even toileting, which is a little embarrassing for a 50 year old.

You may not be able to go back to your job or business, I highly recommend getting counselling as such a huge change in your life will take some talking and working through. You will need to Hope for the best while planning for the worst, in that you may well believe that you will fully recover – good. Meanwhile, get the necessary equipment to assist you in living. Take your time relearning things that you have done automatically, without thinking, this is a frustrating time, but you can do it.

You may need some retraining before you can go back to any job. Yes, this is very frustrating too, but you need to do what you need to do. e.g. I was only 49 when I suffered a massive stroke and was left with my left side paralysed, we had 4 teenage children all still living at

Maxwell R Watson

home with us and all in high school, the Disability Support Pension I was eligible for was just NOT paying the bills. So returning to some kind of paid employment was not really an option, I simply had to find a way to work. (Now >10 years post-stroke and retired, I don't know how I worked that job for 5 years, but I did.)

You may or may not be able to drive a car again; there are many aids and adaptations that can be installed, both in a car or in your home, to assist you.

WILL I STILL BE ABLE TO ENJOY SEX?

Yes, there may be some complications. If you are male, you may have some level of impotence, for which you can get help. You may need to be a little creative, but with understanding, love and care there is no reason that you should not lead a fulfilling sex life. If that is impossible don't worry; you will find, as I have come to accept, sex is not everything! Life can go on quite well for you even if that wonderful activity is no longer possible.

DO I BELIEVE EVERYTHING THERAPISTS TELL ME?

No, absolutely not! They only know what is considered "normal" over a given number of cases. They do not know you or your ability to fight and recover. A personal example:

An Occupational Therapist was trying to convince me to get a special one-handed keyboard for a computer – I steadfastly refused.

My reasoning was simple; "At that time I had been using computers for over 25 years, I am fairly good with computers, but I need to be able to sit and use any computer and not be limited to using a "special" keyboard." As soon as I was released from the rehabilitation hospital I began the process of re-educating myself in computer usage. I quickly found that having the keyboard at a 45 degree angle to my chair made one-handed typing much easier and created a lot less wrist strain than having the keyboard in a "normal" parallel position. (There are specially designed one-handed keyboards if required. Go to http://www.frogpad.com/ image below)

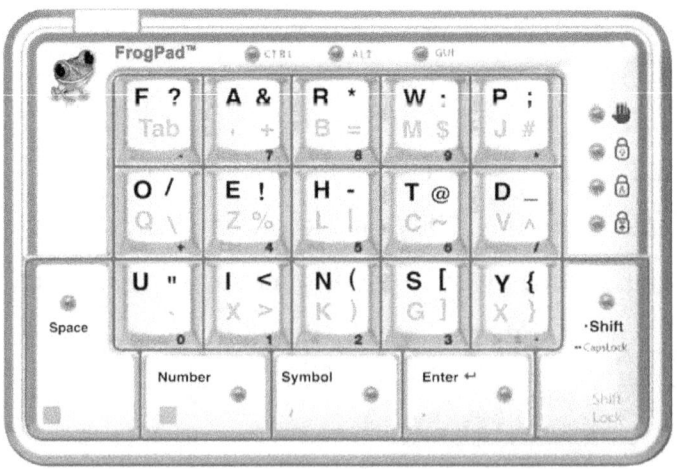

In fact this booklet was written on a standard Apple MacBook Pro and edited on a standard desktop computer using Windows.

WILL I EVER BE "NORMAL" AGAIN?

No-one can answer that question! I'm sorry to be the one to tell you that. If indeed "normal" means anything anyway. You will certainly need to make some life changes, even if your recovery appears to be 100%. You had a stroke – it is not a funny thing that you now live with an ABI. Getting fit, loosing weight, etc. are all important aspects of life that you may need to address. Do it. If you have been a workaholic, then that **MUST** be addressed; e.g. I was a workaholic for many, years; decades infact. It was a contributing factor to my stroke. Get over it, get help, see a counsellor or a life coach, but stop being a workaholic. If you are reading this and have not had a stroke but can relate to this paragraph, do anything whatsoever to avoid having a stroke; tell your overweight work colleagues to get a handle on their weight. I repeat Do ANYTHING TO AVOID A STROKE.

If you have never been a person of faith, then explore your spirituality, it is a fact that people with a strong faith live longer and more contented & fulfilled lives than people with no religious faith. If you have no one you feel comfortable in asking about spirituality, contact me and I will put you in touch with someone near you that will help (regardless of where you are in the world); my email address is located on the title page.

I personally believe the most import attitude to embrace is for you to be totally and completely determined to never, never, never give up. I believe this so much I had it tattooed on my arm, to be my daily reminder.

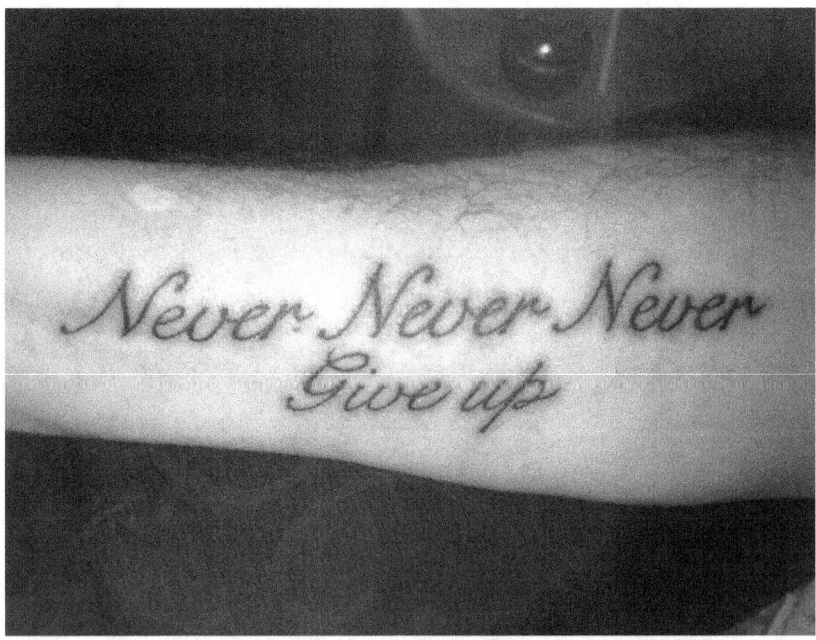

This way, I read my own motto every day: Never, Never, Never Give up!

Understand that you could well experience sea-sawing emotions, even despair of your situation; my emotions were certainly changed due to my stroke. I cry much more easily now and I sometimes feel embarrassed that a story told in church or a movie makes me cry. Keep focused; life is worth living; you were not meant to die. If I had not survived my stroke I would not have seen each of my children graduate high school, would not have witnessed my eldest daughter graduate with her Degree, I would not have walked (I usually say hobbled) two of my girls down the isle at their weddings and I would have never know my Granddaughter Zoe or Grandson Kenan. Do not think that life is not worth living – because it is so very much worth it. It is vital that you seek out the help you need.

ON DOCTORS/THERAPISTS AND COUNSELLORS

Not every doctor, therapist or counsellor will necessarily be the right one for you. I changed my GP after being at that particular practice for 20 years because I felt he was not doing the best a G.P. could or should do for me.

The same goes for Therapists and counsellors. There are varying kinds of counselling and approaches you may find that the first one you see is not necessarily the best option. Do not be afraid to say I want to see someone else. I do know that if you do not address frustration and anger you feel that it will lead to serious problems. But these are battles that can be won.

WHAT WILL MY PARTNER DO?

The secret in continuing to live life well is having a dedicated carer/partner, in my case my amazing wife of 34+ years, Christine, to say she is amazing is a gross understatement. Hyowever, I lack the vocabulary to put into words how amazing she really is. She cares for me in every way. She is patient, reassuring and most importantly she encourages me every step of the way. Even as I am about to get an electric wheelchair, my OT thinks it's time, she has that special ability to see the positives and reassures me that it will be OK and it has been good.

WHAT HELP IS AVAILABLE TO ME?

There is a huge amount of help available, starting with your local General Practitioner. He or she should be able to handle any medical issues or problems you encounter. Confide in him/her, as this relationship will be vital for you in the future.

Therapy on an ongoing basis maybe of benefit to you, or you may get to a point where it is no longer helping you to go forward and you decide to stop going. Again, this is your decision. Do not stop making decisions for yourself, just be sensible – there may well be times when you need to allow your "significant other" to make decisions for you. An example: I suffered a deep and very dark depression; during that time, I had to allow my wife to make some of the more important decisions as I was most definitely unstable.

Another issue is my ABI has meant my hearing has virtually disappeared, to the point that I now have to wear two hearing aides, with which I have a love/hate relationship. I also cannot process complex questions. At some recent medical appointments, I have to allow my wife to do most of the answering of questions, make the decisions, and fill me in later.

Special Note: If you are reading this on behalf of a stroke survivor and their ability to speak has been damaged. Please do not despair, there are ways to learn to communicate again, you just need to keep knocking on doors until you find the right one.

There are many return to work agencies, I suggest you begin with the one your therapist recommends. In Australia that is usually The Commonwealth Rehabilitation Service... The Brain Injury Association is also extremely helpful and I would very highly recommend you visit www.biansw.org.au and or www.brainfacts.org/ and read everything on that site to help you help yourself or your loved one. I'm sure in your country there are similar agencies ask your OT and GP to refer you.

There are numerous disability-focused agencies that can and will help you. Begin by asking your GP, your local Council should have a list or get a friend to do an Internet search of what is available in your area. Never be backward in coming forward to someone to ask.

A few **MUSTS** in closing: You Must:

- Have a positive attitude
- Choose happiness

- Have your medical needs correctly met. This may mean you have to become the like the squeaky wheel in need of oil.
- Make goals
- Set priorities
- Have sub aims to reach each goal. Step by step; baby steps are quite OK.
- Remember above all else:

Never, Never, Never Give Up

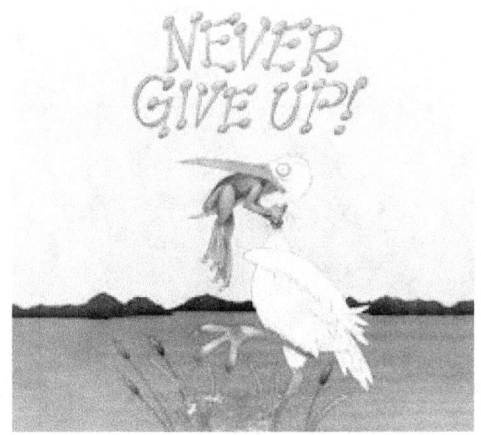

About the Author

I have been through many transitions in life.

I began work at the age of 13 stacking the shelves of a grocery store (this was before supermarkets). I also delivered Telegrams & sewed and laid carpet; all prior to becoming a tradesman electrician, a trade I hated. I eventually grew sideways and went into the professional sound industry, where I became a manager; holding a middle management position. Seeing no future and with my heart on the things of God, I went to study at the Churches of Christ Theological College in New South Wales, Australia, where I eventually earned a Bachelor of Theology degree. After over ten years of both study and ministry, I went to work under the banner of The Foursquare Gospel Church of Australia as both Pastor and School Chaplin.

I married Christine, in 1980, and together they have 4 now adult children, two sons-in-law and two grandchildren.

Again, there was to be yet another transition; I resigned after 7 years at Mt Druitt, a tough area of Western Sydney, I left pastoral ministry and went to run the humanitarian project Operation Christmas Child for Samaritans Purse Australia; it was while I was on an assignment in Cambodia in May 2004, I suffered a massive stroke. Full recovery did not happen, and I was left with Left-side Hemiplegia; meaning my left side is paralysed. I managed to gain a couple of part-time administration jobs; but have most recently concentrated my knowledge and talents to writing. In order to encourage and teach "the church" I love.

My books include:
So You Had a Stroke (a free eBook)
Confronted by Poverty on a 1st Mission Trip
The Collected Short Stories and Verse
Lessons in Life from the Life of Abraham
Life is for Living (a journey through Ecclesiastes)
Living in Christian Joy(a journey through Philippians)
Christianity 101
Another look at Psalm23
The Minor Prophets

They are all available as eBooks or printed books via amazon.com

Please if you even just want to have an email chat I'm available via email or Facebook.

www.ingramcontent.com/pod-product-compliance
Lightning Source LLC
Chambersburg PA
CBHW071349310526
45790CB00018B/1401